indian head

massage

in essence

Mary Dalgleish & Lesley Hart

Series Editor: Nicola Jenkins

Hodder Arnold

A MEMBER OF THE HODDER HEADLINE GROUP

Orders: please contact Bookpoint Ltd, 130 Milton Park, Abingdon, Oxon OX14 4SB. Telephone: (44) 01235 827720. Fax: (44) 01235 400454. Lines are open from 9.00 - 5.00, Monday to Saturday, with a 24 hour message answering service. You can also order through our website www.hoddereducation.co.uk

If you have any comments to make about this, or any of our other titles, please send them to educationenquiries@hodder.co.uk

British Library Cataloguing in Publication Data
A catalogue record for this title is available from the British Library

ISBN: 978 0 340 94165 2

This Edition Published 2007
Impression number   10 9 8 7 6 5 4 3 2 1
Year   2010   2009   2008   2007

Hodder Headline's policy is to use papers that are natural, renewable and recyclable products and made from wood grown in sustainable forests. The logging and manufacturing processes are expected to conform to the environmental regulations of the country of origin.

The information given in this book is not intended as a replacement for medical advice and should not be used for diagnosis or treatment of any medical condition.

Cover photo by Carl Drury
Artwork by Oxford Designers and Illustrators

Typeset by Servis Filmsetting Ltd, Manchester
Printed in Great Britain by CPI Bath